Between Heartbeats and Algorithms

Reclaiming What Matters in Healthcare

Devjit Roy, MD, MAS, MSPC, CPE, CMD, CHCQM, FHM, FAAFP, LSSBB

Foreword by Peter Angood, MD

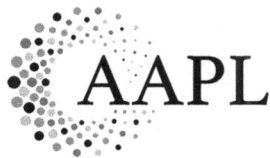

AAPL

Published by **American Association for Physician Leadership, Inc.**
PO Box 96503 | BMB 97493 | Washington, DC 20090-6503

Website: www.physicianleaders.org

AAPL books are available at special quantity discounts to use as premiums and sales promotions, or for use in corporate training programs. For more information, please write to Special Sales at journal@physicianleaders.org

This publication is designed to provide general information and is sold with the understanding that neither the author nor the publisher is engaged in rendering legal, accounting, ethical, or clinical advice. If legal or other expert advice is required, the services of a competent professional person should be sought.

13   8 7 6 5 4 3 2 1

Copyedited, typeset, indexed, and printed in the United States of America

PUBLISHER
Nancy Collins

PRODUCTION MANAGER
Jennifer Weiss

DESIGN & LAYOUT
Carter Publishing Studio

COPYEDITOR
Patricia George

For my wife, my children, my family, my friends,
and my patients — thank you for teaching me, grounding me,
and walking beside me through every step of this journey.

This book is for you.

TABLE OF CONTENTS

About the Author

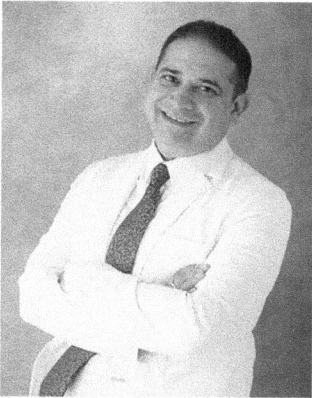

Devjit Roy, MD, MAS, MSPC, LSSBB, FAAFP, FHM, CHCQM, CPE, CMD, is a physician executive and practicing clinician dedicated to advancing rural healthcare. He serves as chief medical officer, chief medical informatics officer, vice president of medical affairs, and medical director for post-acute care at Nathan Littauer Hospital in upstate New York. He is also a board member at Mountain Valley Hospice and co-president of Fulmont Medical PC, a joint venture uniting two rural hospitals.

Dr. Roy's leadership emphasizes integrating innovation with compassion, driving quality improvement, and fostering interdisciplinary collaboration to strengthen patient outcomes across hospital, nursing home, and clinic settings. His clinical practice spans hospital medicine, palliative care, and post-acute care, and he continues to provide direct bedside care while leading organizational transformation.

He is board certified in Family Medicine, Hospital Medicine, Palliative and Hospice Medicine, Lifestyle Medicine, Obesity Medicine, and Quality and Utilization. He also holds master's degrees in Population Health and in Palliative Care.

Since beginning his medical journey in 2009, Dr. Roy has cared for tens of thousands of patients, guided by the belief that every patient has a story worth listening to. His work reflects a focus on presence, curiosity, and humanity in medicine, alongside a commitment to operational excellence and digital equity.

Outside of medicine, he is a teacher, coach, and advocate for physician wellness. He lives in upstate New York with his wife, also a physician, their two young children, and two dogs. He finds renewal in music, martial arts, soccer, and quiet moments with family.

Foreword

THE CRAFT OF NARRATIVE MEDICINE continues to evolve, highlighting how clinicians of all types grapple with the complexities of their chosen professions in this era of healthcare. Patients allow us the privilege of intimacy with their lives, often followed by a subsequent outpouring of gratitude and appreciation that comes from helping them become healthier. And then, occasionally, there are the contrasting circumstances that must be confronted when the inevitable inadequacies of patient care outcomes occur.

In both circumstances, there is a related emotional component that clinicians may or may not be comfortable recognizing or admitting to themselves, let alone with others.

The paradox of clinical healthcare professions is that the people drawn to these professions are typically kind, caring, and compassionate people who care deeply about helping others; however, this altruistic driving force can become difficult to maintain, given the volume of patients cared for during a career and the often-tragic outcomes or patient circumstances they may witness over time.

We must each learn how best to navigate these personal journeys. And at times, it is a tough path to follow. *Between Heartbeats and Algorithms: Reclaiming What Matters in Healthcare* is a beautiful example of narrative medicine. Devjit Roy draws deeply from his personal clinical and emotional experiences in a fashion designed to stir the reader's compassion, empathy, and altruism.

All clinicians have a multitude of clinical stories to tell and memories to share, and Dr. Roy challenges us not to simply bury them within our memory banks. Rather, he dares us to learn from these experiences, to capture their essence of humanity, and to use them to not only help us, but to benefit others as well.

As Dr. Roy describes, "This book is my attempt to … reflect on the spaces where real healing happens … to grow, to learn from story, and to keep myself honest — to preserve our shared humanity in a system that sometimes feels like it's forgetting it."

Drawing on his experiences caring for approximately 50,000 patients, he profiles 15 clinical situations that profoundly affected his views toward medicine and life in general. His storytelling is crafted in a way that resonates with all clinicians, and his writing style is both engaging and reflective.

More importantly, his messages at the end of each story are designed to help readers recognize the emotional connection we all share with our patients and create moments of pause that we can use to better manage ourselves moving forward.

The moments of pause created while I read through this book actually took me down a path of reflection on my own clinical journey as a trauma (acute care) surgeon. Over my clinical time, I performed around 20,000–25,000 trauma resuscitations (typical 10% mortality rate), managed more than 100,000 ICU patients (typical 15% mortality rate), and was involved with 10,000–12,000 end-of-life discussions. No, I don't remember all those cases, but there are a few that still stand out. And I realize now that I should have taken more time to process my own emotions during that time.

Not paying adequate attention to the emotional turmoil and related mental health challenges in the clinical disciplines is now recognized as a contributing factor in compassion fatigue and burnout in the healthcare workforce. Recognizing this insidious erosion of our innate traits of benevolence and compassion is critically important for the betterment of the profession now and for the future.

Fortunately, the topic of burnout has reached a level of general awareness and a multitude of resources are now available as our industry better navigates the complexity of these issues.

But this book does not dwell on the difficult side of clinical care! It is a beautiful collection of poignant, heartfelt stories that anchor the reader back to the reason clinicians choose to devote themselves to the privileged professions of helping others. This book is about helping us to reimagine and recognize the beauty and pleasure of being a healthcare professional. It also challenges us to empower ourselves to ensure none of us forgets about the humanity in healthcare.

This is also a book that clinicians should share with their families and friends, for it will provide patients and the public with deeper insights into how they, themselves, influence physician-patient interactions and how they might better interact with their clinical providers going forward.

The core of every clinical interaction is the deep personal and emotional connections made between the humans who are each trying to make their lives, and the lives of others, better through kindness, caring, and gratitude for one another.

This is a must-read book for anyone involved with healthcare, regardless of whether they are on the giving or the receiving side of the system. You will feel enriched and reassured that humanism is thriving in healthcare, and that many are invested in making sure it is maintained. Enjoy your read and the moments of pause it creates.

Peter Angood, MD
American Association for Physician Leadership
www.physicianleaders.org
October 2025

PROLOGUE

A Life Returned

*The ICU lights were dimmed, the way we kept them at night
to mimic sleep. But sleep was long gone — for all of us.*

HE WAS 42, A FATHER OF TWO, with both end-stage liver disease and renal failure. His skin had turned a dusky yellow. His body loop was swollen with fluid. Machines hummed quietly around him, managing what his own organs could no longer do. Each day, we stabilized one thing only to see another start to fail. He was teetering at the edge, held up by sheer will, the dedication of a care team, and hope that sometimes felt painfully thin.

We knew time was running out. We were honest with the family. "He may not survive the week," I remember saying. Still, they held on. So did we. Dialysis continued. Nutrition was optimized. Conversations turned into coordination. Transplant evaluations. Ethical discussions. Nightly chart reviews that became personal rituals.

And then the call came — a liver was available.

Even then, we weren't sure he'd survive the surgery. The odds were against him. But he did. He survived. Slowly, he started to recover. He left the ICU, then the hospital. We celebrated quietly — cautiously — as we often do in medicine, before moving on to the next critical patient, the next crisis, the next season.

Nearly a year later, I saw him again. It was a busy afternoon at the mall, and I almost walked right past him.

He looked vibrant. Laughing, pushing a stroller, wearing a baseball cap, and holding his wife's hand. He looked like any other dad enjoying a weekend with his family. When he stopped me with a smile and said, "Hey, doc," I hesitated.

I didn't recognize him.

There was a moment of silence — just long enough to feel the weight of it. I was embarrassed. I searched his face, trying to place him, to recall where our paths had crossed. And then, like a slow rush of memory crashing through the fog of time and hospital gowns, it hit me.

This was *him*.

The man I had once watched hover at the edge of life. The man whose family we had gently prepared for goodbye. The man who — against every expectation — got a second chance.

I stood there, speechless. Overwhelmed.

Not just by the transformation, but by the quiet power of seeing him like this. Alive. Thriving. Ordinary in the most extraordinary way.

What struck me wasn't just that he had survived. It was that he had *returned*. To life. To fatherhood. To normalcy. And that perhaps, beneath all the protocols and treatment plans, that's what we're really fighting for in medicine: not just more days, but more *life*. A trip to the mall. A child's laughter. A second chance.

Medicine can be heavy. We don't always get outcomes like this. But once in a while, a patient reminds you why the work matters — why presence matters — why showing up every day, even in the most hopeless moments, is worth it.

This book is a collection of those reminders. Stories of resilience, uncertainty, and grace. Not all of them end like his. But every one of them changed me. These are the stories I carry. The ones that teach. The ones that stay.

The ones that live quietly between heartbeats.

INTRODUCTION

Why These Stories Matter

I didn't set out to write a book. I was just trying to make sense of it all.

AFTER YEARS AS A DIRECT PRIMARY CARE PROVIDER, a hospitalist, and a palliative care physician, I found myself returning to certain patient stories — not because they were dramatic or rare, but because they stuck with me. They were ordinary moments that revealed something essential: about healing, about suffering, about what it means to really see someone.

Medicine has changed so much in the years I've been practicing. The science has advanced, the technology has exploded, and we have more data than ever. But with each advancement, something else has crept in — layers of complexity that now sit between the patient and the provider. Prior authorizations. Documentation requirements. EMR clicks. Third-party administrators. Corporate protocols. What used to be a sacred space between two people — a clinician and a patient — is now crowded with intermediaries.

And it's not just frustrating, it's disorienting. For providers, it means more time checking boxes and less time listening. For patients, it means delays, confusion, and a sense that they're being processed instead of cared for.

In my career, I've cared for more than **50,000 people,** each with their own story, their own struggle, their own heartbeat. But this book isn't about 50,000 patients. It's about **15.** Fifteen people whose lives intersected with mine in ways I couldn't ignore. Fifteen stories that changed how I practice medicine, how I lead, and how I live.

In the world of healthcare operations, we often speak in terms of *value-added* versus *non-value-added* work. Value-added work is what's billable — coded visits, procedures, diagnostics — the parts of care tied directly to reimbursement. It's what the system is built to measure and reward. But then there's non-value-added work: the time spent calling families, coordinating with case managers, listening to a patient cry at 2 a.m., or sitting quietly at the bedside during the final moments of life.

That work doesn't generate relative value units (RVUs). It doesn't show up on performance dashboards. But it's necessary. It's medicine.

And as our system pushes toward standardization, automation, and efficiency — checklists and protocols and AI-generated note templates — we risk losing the very soul of our profession. The art of medicine. The judgment. The listening. The moments that can't be protocolized, but are no less vital.

This book is my attempt to hold on to those moments. To reflect on the spaces where real healing happens — not just in the procedures we bill for, but in the care we offer when no one's watching. It's a reminder that behind every order set and metric is a person. And behind every provider is someone trying to do the right thing in a system that doesn't always make it easy.

I wrote this book to grow, to learn from the story, and to keep myself honest. But more importantly, I wrote it to empower others — especially those working in healthcare — to preserve our shared humanity in a system that sometimes feels like it's forgetting it.

So whether you're a provider, a caregiver, a patient, or simply someone trying to make sense of the world, we all live in the spaces between heartbeats. And that's where the meaning lives.

Part 1

Remembering Humanity

∞

Where the journey begins —
not with knowing, but with noticing.

CHAPTER 1

Listen First – The Power of Bearing Witness

Lesson: *Listening is not a passive act; it is a clinical tool, a diagnostic lens, and a moral responsibility. Sometimes the most powerful medicine is presence.*

THE EMERGENCY DEPARTMENT HAD ALREADY CALLED TWICE. "Sepsis, altered mental status, history of cancer," they said. "She's not very responsive." A familiar handoff in an unfamiliar world — another patient in crisis, another decision to be made before we knew the whole story.

Mrs. K arrived just before shift change — frail, pale, with sunken cheeks and skin like rice paper. The admitting note said she was 81, but the last year had aged her more than any birthday could. The nurse was already hanging antibiotics as I entered the room.

Her name had a familiar ring to it. I scanned the chart. Atrial fibrillation. COPD. Heart failure. Stage III cancer, diagnosed just four months ago. She had been undergoing chemotherapy, and I could see the toll it had taken even before reading the notes: cachectic frame, missing hair beneath the scarf tied around her head, and the unmistakable look of exhaustion in her eyes.

The intern rattled off the vitals and lab results. "Febrile to 102.9, MAP in the 50s, white count 24. We're thinking the source is the port. She's a full code. Family's on their way in."

As they moved on to the next task, I pulled up a chair and sat by her bed. She was awake, but barely. Her breathing shallow, her mouth dry, her eyes clouded — but alert. There was a presence there, beneath the fatigue.

She looked at me. I asked if she was in pain.

"A little," she said, her voice weak but deliberate. "But that's not the worst of it."

I paused. "What is the worst of it?"

She looked off toward the ceiling for a moment. "Being here."

And then, as if she'd been holding it in for weeks, it came tumbling out.

A Quiet Life, and a Long Year

Mrs. K had lived in a small town in Wyoming her whole life. She and her husband had been married for 52 years, and they had raised three children: Lisa, Leslie, and James. They'd had a quiet, rooted life — simple but full — anchored by family dinners, weekend drives, and a shared love of gardening. She spoke about her husband with the reverence reserved for lifelong partners. "After he died," she said, "I stopped wanting much of anything."

He had passed away eight months ago. Since then, Mrs. K's world had become smaller. Her energy, dulled by grief and chemotherapy, was spent mostly in a recliner by the living room window. "I used to walk down the block and back," she said. "Now I don't even go to the porch." Food lost its taste. Music made her cry. Visitors came less often. "I have my home health aide and my daughter," she said. "That's enough."

Her oldest daughter, Lisa, lived nearby and had become her primary caregiver. She was the one managing medications, coordinating appointments, and seeing the daily toll of both the disease and the treatment. Her daughter Leslie, who lived in California, and her son James, who lived in Florida, had not been involved in the same way.

There had been a long-standing estrangement between Leslie and James — one that began during their father's funeral and solidified over disagreements about their mother's care. In truth, they hadn't seen each other in over 15 years. A distance that had once been geographic had grown into silence. Now, facing their mother's decline, the weight of those lost years hung heavily between them. Lisa had stayed neutral, but privately, she supported her mother's wish to stop treatment. "She's been through enough," Lisa had told me later. "But I didn't want to be the one to make that call — not with everything going on between them."

The Turning Point

I sat by Mrs. K's side a while longer. She talked slowly, her voice growing softer. "I didn't want the chemo," she said. "But I did it for them. For the kids. I didn't want to be the one to let go."

I asked her a simple question: "What would you want, if this were entirely your choice?"

She closed her eyes for a moment. "To go home. To sit in my chair. Maybe hear the wind chimes one more time."

When Lisa arrived at the hospital later that afternoon, I sat with both of them. I shared what her mother had said, and to my surprise, Lisa didn't flinch.

"She's been telling me this for weeks," Lisa said gently. "I just didn't know if anyone else would listen."

We arranged a family meeting. Leslie and James joined by phone. The conversation was fragile, emotional, and tense. Leslie asked about second opinions. James asked what else we hadn't tried. Lisa stayed quiet at first, then gently said, "Mom is tired. She doesn't want more. She wants peace."

Something in her voice broke the silence. Eventually, there was an understanding — a shared grief, spoken from different corners of the country. The siblings agreed to come.

And they did.

The next day, Leslie flew in from California. James arrived from Florida shortly after. For the first time in over 15 years, the three siblings sat in the same room.

The last 48 hours of Mrs. K's life were sacred. She was lucid at times, comfortable throughout. She held each of their hands. Lisa managed her medications. Leslie brought her fresh flowers. James read her favorite poem. They shared old stories, laughter through tears, and soft apologies.

And perhaps most important of all, Leslie and James reconciled. The weight of grief softened the edge of pride. The disagreements faded into gratitude for the chance to be together. In the final hours of their mother's life, they began to mend something broken long before her illness began.

Mrs. K passed away peacefully two days later. No alarms. No machines. Just breath, and then stillness.

Reflection: The Lesson She Taught Me

In the practice of medicine, we often default to doing. Intervening.

Escalating. Continuing treatment. And in the flurry of orders and labs and alarms, we can forget that sometimes the most important thing we can do is sit still and listen.

Mrs. K reminded me that patients do not fear death as much as they fear dying the wrong way — disconnected, unheard, and far from what they would have chosen. Her quiet clarity cut through the noise of family conflict, physician recommendations, and institutional momentum. What she needed was not more medicine. She needed someone to ask, "What matters now?"

And then to act on the answer.

Closing Thought

Listening is not a passive act. In healthcare, it is a clinical tool, a diagnostic lens, and a moral responsibility. To bear witness to suffering without rushing to fix it is one of the hardest — and most human — things we can do.

For Mrs. K, it made all the difference.

CHAPTER 2

The Ones Who Stayed, The Ones Who Didn't

Lesson: *Knowing what kind of work you are meant to do means also knowing what kind you are not. There is courage in showing up — and there is wisdom in stepping back.*

IT WAS MY THIRD NIGHT IN A ROW on call in a high-risk pediatric hospital. I had already stopped counting the hours. The halls felt quieter at night, but never calmer. The hum of incubators, the sudden bursts of alarms, the whispered updates — it all lived under a different kind of gravity when the patients were just hours or days old.

That week, five newborns were born not breathing.

Five.

Each a different story. Each a beginning that teetered on the edge of an end.

Three of those babies survived. Two did not.

I remember each of them in different ways, but the last one — that fifth baby — stayed with me in a way I didn't expect. It was near the end of my call week, and I was already emotionally threadbare.

We were called to the delivery room for a high-risk labor, and something in the air already felt heavy. The baby emerged limp, cyanotic, not breathing. Her Apgar score was 0 at one minute.

We began neonatal resuscitation immediately.

Warmed blankets. Stimulation. Bag-mask ventilation. Intubation. Chest compressions. Epinephrine. Repeat. Check for heart tones. Still nothing.

Minute after minute passed. Twenty. Thirty. Forty. Her body was purple. We coded her for nearly an hour. And for most of that time, it felt like we were trying to hold onto a soul already halfway gone.

But then, a flicker.

A faint heart rate.

We kept going.

She took a breath. Then another.

She cried.

Color returned to her skin. Her limbs moved. We stabilized her. Transferred her to the NICU. And waited.

That night, I didn't exhale until hours later. After all the sadness of the previous days — after watching two other newborns slip away — this tiny life had come back.

And somehow, despite everything she endured in that first hour, she survived. And not just survived — she thrived. Over the following months, she grew into a healthy baby girl with no neurological deficits, no developmental delays. She came back from the brink. She was whole.

The Emotional Aftermath

That week broke something open in me.

I didn't cry at work. I didn't have time. But when I got home, when the adrenaline wore off and the quiet settled in, the grief showed up in my dreams.

I dreamt of the babies who didn't make it. Not as ghosts or symbols — but as moments. I'd hear the monitors. I'd see the stillness. I'd feel the hopeless rhythm of compressions without a response.

It wasn't just grief. It was a deep, personal knowing: This wasn't my work.

Learning What Wasn't Mine

I have immense respect for pediatricians — for those who stay in those NICUs, who walk with families through the most vulnerable hours of life. That week showed me that I could be part of it when I had to. I could act. I could help.

But I also learned I wasn't built to stay.

In my family medicine residency, I already felt drawn toward adult medicine — toward hospital care, acute and chronic illness, and the quiet depth of palliative conversations. I found my presence was most helpful in complexity, in long-term relationships, in witnessing stories unfold. Pediatrics — and especially neonatal trauma — asked something of my spirit that I couldn't give over and over again.

That doesn't make it less important. It makes it sacred, and it makes the discernment even more vital.

Reflection: What They Taught Me

Those newborns, in their brief and fragile lives, taught me about the weight of medicine and the importance of knowing my own boundaries.

They taught me that part of becoming a physician is learning not only what you're good at, but what you're meant for.

I also learned that I could still find meaning in this space — not in resuscitating babies, but in being present for families navigating the unimaginable. In sitting with a mother whose child didn't make it. In holding space for grief when there are no more interventions to offer.

And I'll never forget that last baby.

She reminded me that sometimes, the body remembers how to fight, even when the odds say otherwise. That medicine can still hold mystery. That light can return even after an hour in the dark.

Closing Thought

That week changed me. Not because I couldn't save them all, but because I realized I wasn't meant to carry every kind of loss. And that's okay.

The last baby taught me that even when everything looks gone, there's still a chance for return. Her fight gave me one too.

She reminded me that medicine isn't only about what you can do — it's about what you're called to do. And sometimes, the most courageous choice is to step away from what you're good at so you can serve fully where you're meant to be.

Her story stays with me. As do all the others. And so does the lesson: To practice medicine with heart, we must know our own.

CHAPTER 3

We Treat More Than Organs

Lesson: Healthcare is often fragmented — split between specialists, systems, and silos. Treating the whole person means bringing those fragments back together to restore coherence, clarity, and trust.

HE CAME IN ON A TUESDAY AFTERNOON, brought in by his daughter after another episode of confusion. Mr. R was 64 years old and already a veteran of the hospital system. This was his third admission in six weeks.

Diabetes, COPD, Stage 3 chronic kidney disease, heart failure with reduced ejection fraction, peripheral neuropathy, GERD, depression. His chart read like a textbook index. The medication list stretched over a page and a half. Eighteen prescriptions. Two inhalers. A weekly injection. Supplements. A sliding-scale insulin regimen. He was seeing seven different specialists.

No one could quite agree on what the problem was this time. His daughter said he'd become confused and sleepy again. The nephrologist thought it was a volume issue. The cardiologist suspected beta-blocker toxicity. Endocrinology suggested hypoglycemia. The notes were thorough. The labs were trending. The teams were engaged. But the patient was adrift.

When I walked into his room, he was staring at the ceiling, arms folded over his chest. "I'm tired," he said, without looking at me.

"Tired like sleepy, or tired like done?" I asked.

He turned to me then. "Both."

A Life in Pieces

His daughter, Rachel, sat by the window with a bag of carefully organized paperwork — printouts of clinic notes, bottles of medications, a yellow legal pad filled with questions. She was his caregiver, his advocate, his surrogate for appointments he no longer had the energy to attend.

Before his health began to decline, Mr. R had led an extraordinarily full and disciplined life. He worked two jobs: one as a respected mathematics professor at a local university, and the other as a successful day trader. He had accumulated millions of dollars through decades of discipline and strategy. His mornings began with exercise. He played chess competitively, completed advanced sudoku puzzles, cooked like a trained chef, and played classical piano by ear.

But when his illness journey began, his world started to fragment. First, it was fatigue and forgetfulness. Then came the hospitalizations, the referrals, the changes in medications.

He found himself lost in a maze of healthcare — juggling doctor visits, admissions, acute and subacute rehab stays in nursing facilities, and long calls with insurance companies. He bounced between pharmacies, specialists, naturopaths, and chiropractors, all offering partial answers but no clear direction.

"Every doctor is telling us something different," Rachel said. "They mean well, but no one talks to each other. And every time we go to one, the meds change. He used to be sharp. Now, he's afraid to take anything."

Rachel had been managing his care full-time since her mother died the year prior. Her own life — a job in tech, two young kids — had slowly shrunk around her father's needs. She wasn't angry, just worn down. "I just want one person to look at the whole picture," she said.

The Turning Point

Mr. R was admitted under my care as the treating hospitalist with a constellation of symptoms: worsening confusion, persistent nausea and vomiting, inability to tolerate oral intake, acute pancreatitis, and renal failure. The pancreatitis was unexpected; he wasn't a drinker, and he had no history of gallstones or gallbladder issues. After reviewing his medications, we began to suspect the pancreatitis was drug-induced.

I sat down with the chart and the med list that night. It took almost an hour to reconcile it all. There were duplications. Conflicts. Medications prescribed for side effects caused by other medications. A drug the cardiologist started last month that nephrology had discontinued two weeks later. An insulin dose lowered by endocrinology but not communicated to his primary.

I arranged a multidisciplinary meeting that included all of his specialists. We brought together the cardiologist, nephrologist, pulmonologist, endocrinologist, psychiatrist, and pharmacist — all in the same room, along with me, the patient, and Rachel. We walked through every medication, every symptom, every unresolved question. Just getting everyone on the same page made all the difference.

By the end of that visit, his medication list was reduced from 18 to just 4. Of those four, Mr. R expressed that he didn't want to continue one due to unwanted side effects. We honored his preference.

With close monitoring of his bloodwork, frequent follow-ups, and daily observation by Rachel, Mr. R was transformed within a week. His energy returned. His mental clarity improved. The fatigue and fog that had clouded him for months lifted.

We streamlined his care, prioritized symptom control over perfect numbers, and ensured everyone was aligned. The nephrologist backed off a diuretic that had been worsening fatigue. The endocrinologist simplified the insulin regimen. The cardiologist signed off on a more conservative strategy.

By simplifying his medications, looking at side effects, and trialing strategies to determine which medications he actually needed — rather than prescribing medications to treat side effects of other medications — we began to uncover the root cause of his symptoms.

His myriad complaints stemmed from a delayed diagnosis. Once the correct diagnosis was determined and understood, the list of medications was re-evaluated and reduced to just what he truly needed.

The transformation was striking. His confusion lifted. His incontinence improved. His nausea, reflux, dry mouth, and appetite returned to baseline. And with those improvements, something remarkable happened: He went back to hunting and fishing. He returned to the golf course. Activities he hadn't been able to enjoy in two years.

By avoiding premature closure, reviewing everything that had been done by previous physicians and providers, and building my own comprehensive assessment, we were able to reset a hijacked illness journey. Mr. R regained control of his life.

Rachel teared up. "This is the first time I feel like someone sees the whole picture," she said.

Reflection: The Lesson He Taught Me

Mr. R reminded me that we do not treat lab values or scan results — we treat people. People whose lives are shaped not only by illness, but by fear, fatigue, and fractured systems. In our effort to manage diseases, we risk losing sight of the person navigating them.

But there was another, deeper lesson too: In this case, I wasn't only treating Mr. R, I was also treating the doctors involved in his care. Each of them cared deeply, each brought expertise, but none had the full picture. What Mr. R truly needed was a coordinated team, and part of my work became treating the team as if they were a patient — listening, diagnosing the communication gaps, and helping them come together for a shared, patient-centered plan.

Fragmentation is not just a systems issue — it is a human issue. And coherence, when restored, can be healing in itself.

Closing Thought

In medicine, doing more is not always doing better. Sometimes, the most radical act is to pause, zoom out, and ask: *Are we still treating the person, or just their parts?*

Mr. R gave me the answer. And a new way to practice.

Doctors will use the tools they know. If a doctor is a hammer, the patient may be seen as a nail — and some may keep hammering away. But not every patient is a nail. It is important for us to remain humble in the presence of our patients and their stories, and to be curious enough to learn from them. Sometimes the best solution is not another test or prescription — but a difficult conversation.

In this case, the difficult conversation was not just with the patient, but among the experts. It was creating space for six specialists to come together, to listen, and to agree on a plan that made sense for the person they were trying to help. A plan that honored the patient's life — not just their conditions.

CHAPTER 4

What the Chart Doesn't Say

Lesson: Trauma doesn't always show up in a patient's words. Sometimes it lives in behaviors we misinterpret. Compassion begins with asking, not assuming.

SHE CAME IN FOR WEAKNESS.

A 52-year-old woman, married, with one daughter, admitted for evaluation of fatigue, dizziness, and what turned out to be a gastrointestinal bleed. I hadn't met her before, but before I even walked into the room, I already had an image forming in my mind.

The chart told a certain kind of story.

Multiple medication allergies. Noncompliance with prior treatment plans. "Refused labs." "Did not follow up." "Challenging historian." The red flags were everywhere — subtle language, fragmented notes, embedded assumptions. It was all there, and if I'm honest, I felt the bias starting to take shape before I heard her voice.

But then I met her.

And everything I had started to assume began to fall apart.

She was thoughtful. Kind. She asked good questions and listened attentively to my explanations. She expressed gratitude for her husband, who sat quietly in the corner of the room, steady and supportive. She was open, even vulnerable. Nothing about her behavior aligned with the notes I had read.

Still, something felt inconsistent.

I couldn't quite name it, but there was a dissonance between how she presented and how the system had portrayed her. The tone in the documentation didn't match the person in the bed. I held onto that curiosity, even as her clinical course unfolded.

A Hidden Diagnosis

On the third day of her admission, something unexpected happened.

I had gone into the room to explain the need for a colonoscopy. Her hemoglobin had dropped, and the bleeding needed to be localized. As I began describing the procedure — its risks, benefits, and need for sedation — her facial expression went blank. Her posture stiffened. Her hands began to tremble.

Then she slumped forward slightly, and her eyes darted quickly to the left.

My clinical reflexes kicked in.

Was this a seizure?

I began preparing to call a code neuro. I considered reaching for lorazepam. My heart rate climbed as I scanned the situation, trying to decipher whether this was an acute neurological event. I was on the edge of initiating the response.

But then her husband, calm but focused, placed his hand gently on her arm and said:

"Wait. Just give it 15 seconds. It's happening."

I froze, caught between protocol and curiosity.

Exactly 15 seconds later, she sat upright. Her eyes sharpened. Her voice, when she spoke, was lower and firmer. Her entire demeanor shifted. She became alert. Defensive. Suspicious. She looked at me with a steadiness that hadn't been there moments ago.

And she looked different — not physically, but energetically. Her tone, cadence, and posture were no longer the same.

It was not a seizure.

It was a personality switch.

What I had just witnessed was one of her alters — an aggressive, protective identity emerging in response to perceived threat.

I had never seen anything like it. Not in real life. Not in practice. Only in case studies and television portrayals. But this was neither dramatized nor exaggerated. This was deeply real. And I was stunned — not just by the shift, but by how routine it was to her husband.

I could only imagine what it must be like for her — to live with these internal shifts, these protective fragments of self that surfaced without warning.

That moment was my gateway into understanding what dissociative identity disorder truly meant — not as a diagnosis, but as a survival strategy.

A Consult That Changed My Practice

We consulted psychiatry. The psychiatrist who came was calm, steady, and carried a deep understanding of trauma.

She explained DID not as a curiosity, but as a coping mechanism born of intense and prolonged trauma — often beginning in early childhood. She explained that each identity, or "alter," had a role in the patient's psychological survival.

But what she shared next changed my practice.

She introduced me to the framework of trauma-informed care — not just for patients, but for families, and even for ourselves.

"The medical system often retraumatizes people," she said. "When someone doesn't take their meds, or misses appointments, or pushes back on care, it may not be resistance. It may be protection."

That sentence cracked something open for me.

How many times had I seen "noncompliant" in a chart and assumed laziness, neglect, or willful disregard? How many times had I interpreted missed appointments as a sign of apathy, rather than a reflection of survival?

A Shift in My Lens

I began to see her differently. Not just her, but every patient like her.

I began to imagine what trauma might look like without a label. The trauma of poverty. Of abuse. Of racial and gender-based discrimination. Of being misunderstood or dismissed.

And I began to ask better questions.

Instead of "Why didn't you take your medication?" I asked, "What got in the way of taking it?"

Instead of assuming someone didn't care about their health, I asked what else they were carrying.

And over time, that curiosity changed the way I charted. The way I spoke. The way I listened.

Reflection: What She Taught Me

This patient, with her many selves, taught me the power of the story behind the story.

She taught me that the chart is a snapshot, not a full picture. That what's documented is filtered through bias, bandwidth, and what we, as clinicians, choose to write down.

She reminded me that trauma doesn't always scream. Sometimes it hides in behaviors that make no sense to us — until we stop, ask, and make space.

And she reminded me **that trauma-informed care isn't a specialty skill** — it's a mindset. A posture of humility. A clinical stance that says, "I don't know what this person has been through, but I will treat them as if they've been through something hard."

Closing Thought

The chart told one story. She told another. And the truth lived somewhere in between.

She reminded me that we are not here to judge what we don't understand. We are here to listen, to learn, and to approach every patient as someone who might be healing from something we'll never fully see. That one shift — in lens, in language, in presence — might be the most important treatment we offer.

Part II

Surviving
the System

∞

Where the path becomes uncertain and
the work becomes heavier.

CHAPTER 5

When We Didn't Know

Lesson: In uncertainty, we survive through curiosity, humility, and grit. These values carried us through a pandemic — and can carry us through any unknown.

THE FIRST PATIENTS CAME IN DECEMBER 2019. They didn't look like much at first — cases of what we assumed was walking pneumonia. Their chest X-rays showed patchy infiltrates, but their flu tests were negative. RSV: negative. Mycoplasma and sputum cultures: negative. Nothing added up. We didn't know it yet, but COVID-19 had already arrived.

By January, we started to suspect something different was happening. And by March 2020, it was undeniable. Our hospital, like so many others across the country, faced a tidal wave.

As a hospitalist, my typical census was 22 to 24 patients. By the time the surge hit, I was managing 35 to 42 patients per day. Fifty to 60% of them would die within the first few days of admission, and then more would be admitted. It was relentless. It didn't matter if they were 18 or 95, male or female, healthy or burdened by chronic conditions. COVID-19 was indiscriminate in its devastation.

Even when we managed to stabilize a patient enough to discharge them off supplemental oxygen, they would often return within 48 hours — gasping, blue, and in fulminant respiratory failure. Many died on readmission. We didn't know why. We tried everything: steroids, antibiotics, breathing treatments, oxygen, Lasix, albumin. We threw every tool we had at the virus, guided by a mix of instinct, theory, and desperate hope.

Then we discovered the clots.

Pulmonary emboli, strokes, limb ischemia. COVID-19 was not just a respiratory disease; it was a vascular one. Microthrombi were forming throughout the body. We began anticoagulating patients early, and some began to survive the first week. We were starting to learn, but slowly. Painfully. Publicly.

And in the middle of it all was Mr. T.

He was 58 years old, married for 25 years. His wife was one of our own — a hospital employee. He had no chronic illnesses. He didn't smoke, didn't drink. He exercised regularly. He was, by every measure, healthy.

He tested positive for COVID in early April. On hospital day two, he deteriorated rapidly. We intubated him. For 20 days, he remained ventilated, sedated, and paralyzed. When he failed to improve, we performed a tracheostomy and placed a PEG tube. He developed recurrent infections from his Foley catheter and from his tracheostomy. Fevers returned. Still, he didn't wake up.

Sixty days passed.

He remained in what appeared to be a vegetative state. His eyes didn't follow movement. His body didn't respond to pain. There were whispered conversations about withdrawal of care. His wife sat at his bedside every day, unwavering, praying, hoping.

Something about his condition didn't feel final to me. It reminded me of Parkinson's patients I had seen with Locked-In Syndrome. There were moments — fleeting ones — where his eyes seemed too purposeful, his brow too subtly furrowed. He didn't have Parkinson's. He hadn't had a stroke. But something told me there was still someone in there.

I discussed the idea with neurology. We trialed two medications. Two days later, he opened his eyes. Then he tracked movement. Then he began to follow commands.

The team was stunned.

We watched a man who had been nearly written off begin to re-enter his body. His wife cried. The nurses cried. I cried.

He was transferred to rehab and then discharged home. Slowly, he regained strength. He spoke. He laughed. He lived.

The Team: Holding the Line Together

COVID was not just a test of medicine. It was a test of spirit.

Our ER, hospital, and ICU providers, nurses, respiratory therapists, physical, occupational, and speech therapists — the entire clinical team — came together like never before. Even as our own fell ill.

We endured physical exhaustion, the loss of friends and patients, and the suffocating weight of uncertainty. I remember sleeping in my car because I was terrified of infecting my wife. I remember calling families so their loved ones could say goodbye. I remember the silence after each code.

But we showed up. And kept showing up.

Reflection: The Lesson He Taught Me

Mr. T's story taught me that in the face of the unknown, three qualities carried us through: curiosity, humility, and grit.

It was curiosity that kept us asking questions when there were no clear answers. We examined every detail, revisited assumptions, and explored possibilities others may have overlooked. In those early days of COVID, curiosity became a clinical lifeline — it kept us learning, adapting, and pushing boundaries.

It was humility that reminded us how little we truly knew. We had to accept that textbook medicine was not enough. Every decision had to be made with the recognition that we were students of a disease we didn't yet understand. Humility kept us grounded, honest, and open to change.

And most of all, it was grit — the deep, enduring, quiet strength — that carried us forward. The grit of the clinical team, who showed up each day despite trauma and fatigue. The grit of Mr. T's wife, who stayed at his bedside in unwavering faith, even when hope seemed thin. And the grit of Mr. T himself, who fought through silence, through paralysis, and through odds no one thought he could overcome.

These three qualities — curiosity, humility, and grit — became our guideposts. They are what allowed healing to happen, not only in bodies, but in spirits.

Sometimes, not giving up is the treatment. Sometimes, the most powerful thing you can offer isn't certainty — it's your continued presence, your belief, and your will to keep trying.

Closing Thought

In those early weeks of COVID, we thought we knew how the story would end. But Mr. T reminded me that in medicine, and especially in the margins of uncertainty, we must leave space for the unexpected. Not everything can be forecasted. Not every miracle is fiction. Sometimes, not giving up is the treatment.

His recovery was more than clinical — it was a testament to the human spirit. The sheer grit and discipline he showed through months of silence, setbacks, and slow steps forward left an indelible mark on me. If he could find a way to come back from the edge, then surely, I could find the strength to keep going too.

CHAPTER 6

Managing Ourselves
to Help Others

*Lesson: We cannot pour from an empty cup. Physician
wellness isn't a luxury — it is a foundation. If we don't
care for ourselves, we cannot care for others.*

HE WAS 54 YEARS OLD. A respected primary care physician. Over the
course of two decades, he had built a bustling, thriving practice: a loyal
panel of patients, a trusted clinical team, and a reputation for being both
compassionate and efficient. On paper, he was successful. Personally.
Professionally. Financially.

But beneath the surface, the fault lines were forming.

Healthcare was changing. Administrative burdens were rising. Reimbursement was shrinking. Then came the federal mandate for electronic
medical records. His group needed to adopt a new EMR. He led the charge
— negotiated with vendors, customized templates, and trained his team.

But the system was clunky. His partners struggled to adjust. He took on
more to support them — redesigning workflows, troubleshooting, and
cleaning up encounters after hours. He became the EMR lead, the IT help
desk, and the safety net.

Meanwhile, insurance denials started rising. Billing delays worsened.
Patient frustration grew. Staff morale dropped. And through it all, he
pushed himself harder — maintaining patient volume, documentation
accuracy, and his identity as the dependable one.

Until one night, after another 14-hour day, he drove home through a rain-
storm — exhausted. He was struck at an intersection by another vehicle.
Both drivers survived. But he did not walk away unchanged.

Multiple rib fractures. A spinal compression fracture. A complex hip
fracture. He was hospitalized for weeks. In pain for months. And placed
on opioids from day one.

The Descent

The pain was real. So was the medication. But somewhere between surgery and recovery, between sleepless nights and growing despair, the pills stopped being medicine and started being a way to get through the day.

A crutch. A numbing agent. A companion.

Then came the alcohol. At first, it was to help him sleep. Then it became routine. Then necessary.

He missed a meeting. Then a week. Then his license was suspended. His practice fell apart. His marriage followed. And the shame was suffocating.

That's when I met him — as his direct primary care physician.

The Coaching Journey

He was burned out — emotionally, physically, spiritually. The medical system had failed him in some ways. But he also had to confront how he had failed himself.

We didn't begin with medications. We began with trust. Slowly, over time, we built a care plan that didn't just treat his addiction — it helped rebuild his life.

We started small. Daily routines. Sleep hygiene. Morning structure. Movement. Gratitude practice. Reflection. Small, consistent habit changes — so subtle they almost seemed insignificant. But over time, those micro-adjustments added up.

This was the power of coaching: helping someone shape their environment, perception, and mindset just enough to create room for self-healing.

He enrolled in a structured recovery program. Began therapy. Attended peer support groups. And we worked through coaching conversations focused not on reinvention, but realignment.

Over two years, his identity began to shift. He developed insight into his thought patterns, his triggers, his avoidance behaviors. He rebuilt his professional confidence. He got involved in peer support. Eventually, he returned to practice — not in the same specialty, but in a deeper calling: addiction medicine.

He now uses his lived experience to help others who are suffering, ashamed, and afraid. And he does it with compassion few can offer, because he's been there. He's walked through the fire.

The Dishes Metaphor

Through our conversations, I shared with him a metaphor that I've come to live by:

From the time we are toddlers — about two years old — we begin accumulating "emotional dishes." These are the unprocessed experiences of grief, guilt, shame, fear, disappointment, and the quiet lies we tell ourselves to cope.

If you eat a meal and don't clean up afterward, the dishes pile up. If you keep doing that meal after meal, day after day, the sink overflows. Eventually, there are so many dirty dishes, you don't know where to begin. It becomes overwhelming. Paralyzing.

That's what emotional overload feels like.

He embraced the metaphor. After every emotional "meal" — a hard conversation, a setback, a good day — he washed his dishes. Through therapy. Through journaling. Through meditation. Through honest reflection. He built a system not for perfection, but for presence.

And I began doing the same.

Triggers and Tells

Over time, I've also learned that there are early warning signs — *tells* — that signal when I'm starting to spin off course. They're often subtle, easily dismissed in the rush of daily life. But once you begin to notice them, they become invaluable cues to pause, reflect, and reset.

For me, the tells are almost always environmental before they are emotional.

When my car is cluttered.

When my desk is disorganized.

When dishes pile up at home, or I can't find something I need.

When I start showing up late to meetings or overlook a task that was mine to complete.

These small breakdowns aren't random. They are indicators — data points that suggest something deeper is stirring beneath the surface. They're not just signs of being "busy." They're signs of misalignment.

When I notice these tells, I know it's time to course-correct. Sometimes that means meditating. Sometimes it means journaling, walking, or doing something physical to ground myself. Other times, it means stepping back and asking the harder question: *What has triggered me?*

Triggers, I've come to understand, are often rooted in something that feels threatened — something important to us, often below conscious awareness. I use the SCARF model as a framework:

Status – Has something challenged my sense of competence or respect?

Certainty – Am I facing ambiguity that makes me feel unstable?

Autonomy – Do I feel like I've lost control over something I value?

Relatedness – Have I experienced disconnection or exclusion?

Fairness – Has something felt unjust or out of balance?

When any one of these is activated, it can send us into reactive mode — sometimes subtly, sometimes explosively. Recognizing this pattern has helped me shift from reaction to reflection.

The goal isn't to avoid triggers entirely — that's not realistic. It's to *recognize* them early, *understand* what they mean, and *respond* with intention.

We don't have to wait until burnout or breakdown to make a change. Often, the clues are already there — in our calendars, our homes, our behaviors, and our breath. The key is learning to listen.

Owning My Own Story

I'm not above this work. I've burned out. I've had moments when the pager buzzed and I felt nothing but dread. I've questioned my purpose. I've struggled in silence.

And I'm not ashamed to say: I've had a therapist. I've worked with coaches. I've leaned on mentors. These guides have helped me clean my own dishes — sometimes daily, sometimes desperately.

I believe every physician should gain insight and awareness of themselves. Not just when they're in crisis, but as part of their professional and personal growth. Medicine demands so much of us. We owe it to ourselves to build the internal tools to stay whole.

We cannot pour from an empty cup. We cannot give what we don't have. But when we are well — when we are grounded, clear, and present — we can be a source of healing for everyone we meet.

There's a simple truth I return to often: A candle only needs a spark, some wick, and oxygen to burn. If we as physicians can tend to our own flame — protect it, nourish it, and keep it from going out — then we can continue to light the candles of others.

When we put on our own oxygen masks, when we prioritize wellness, insight, and balance, we become beacons. And in doing so, we empower others in their healing and growth — not just through our clinical knowledge, but through our example.

Reflection: What He Taught Me

The physician I worked with taught me that addiction is not a moral failing — it is a coping strategy that outlives its usefulness. It's something any of us can fall into. Food. Sugar. Work. Alcohol. Perfectionism. The list goes on. Every addiction creates its own set of illnesses. The antidote is balance. And balance requires awareness, intention, and ongoing support.

He also taught me that burnout isn't just about exhaustion. It's about disconnection from meaning. From self. From community.

And he reminded me that recovery — real recovery — is possible. But it's not heroic. It's not a single act of will. It's the daily decision to stay present, to be honest, and to reach out for help when you need it.

Closing Thought

All a candle needs is a spark, some wick, and oxygen to burn.

If we tend to our own flame — carefully, honestly, consistently — then we can continue to light the candles of others. When we put on our own oxygen masks, when we cultivate our wellness and clarity, we become beacons.

We become examples. And in doing so, we empower others — not just through our knowledge, but through our presence.

We are not alone. We were never meant to be.

CHAPTER 7

The Weight We Don't See

Lesson: Even those who seem steady may be carrying more than we know. Hidden burdens can break even the strongest among us.

HE WAS 49. A PHYSICIAN. A COLLEAGUE. A FRIEND.

He was one of the good ones — quiet, competent, always kind.

He showed up for his patients, showed up for his team, and never asked for much. His notes were meticulous. His manner, humble. He wasn't flashy. He wasn't loud. He was just… steady. And then, one Monday morning, he was gone.

He died by suicide.

The Shock

None of us saw it coming.

But in the silence that followed his death, the pieces slowly emerged. He had graduated from medical school with over $410,000 in loans. Years later, through capitalized interest and deferrals, the balance had ballooned to $1.8 million. He never missed a payment. He kept working, even when it didn't seem possible.

He was a primary care physician. He didn't own a large home. He drove a modest car. He wasn't in it for prestige. He did it to serve.

He was also a father who kept working to support his children even after his wife left and took the kids in the divorce. He never spoke about it. But he carried it all — child support, living expenses, professional obligations — without complaint.

He also supported his aging parents financially, never mentioning how heavy the load had become. Always polite. Always responsive. Never once showed us the cracks.

Until it was too late.

The Last Time I Saw Him

I remember the day he came into the hospital. Chest pain. Nausea. Light-headedness. He looked tired, but alert. His cardiac workup was unremarkable. His GI consult ruled out ulcers, reflux, and gallbladder issues. Eventually, someone wrote "panic attacks" in the discharge summary. We sent him home with reassurance and follow-up. And then I never saw him again — until I saw his obituary.

It was over a year later. A colleague sent me the link. I clicked, expecting to read of a sudden illness, a tragic accident. But the truth was harder. He had died by suicide.

What I Didn't Know Then

I didn't know about the $1.8 million in loans.

I didn't know about the legal battles over custody.

I didn't know he had stopped seeing friends.

I didn't know he'd quietly withdrawn from his favorite activities.

I didn't know how often he wondered if it would ever get better.

I didn't know — because he never said.

But maybe I should have asked.

The Collateral Damage in Healthcare

What we also don't talk about is this: The trauma of practicing medicine is not always loud, visible, or singular. It is repetitive. Cumulative. Insidious.

Every difficult case, every code blue, every dying child, every grieving family — it leaves a mark. Each one inflicts a tiny bruise on the brain. And over time, the bruises add up.

A boxer steps into the ring and gets hit. Repeated trauma can cause chronic traumatic encephalopathy or pugilistic Parkinson's. It's visible. We study it. We track it.

But what about the ER doctor who absorbs the cries of a mother whose child won't wake up? What about the ICU nurse who watches a patient die after a futile resuscitation, then scrubs up and enters the next room like nothing happened? What about the hospitalist who breaks the news — again — that there's nothing more we can do?

These are hits, too. Hits to the soul. Hits to the limbic system. Hits to our sense of self.

We don't know what that trauma does to the human brain long term. But it changes us. Quietly. Permanently. And unlike the boxer, there's no audience, no bell, no trainers on the sideline to call the match when we've taken too many blows.

There is no MRI for moral injury. There is no ICD-10 code for the cost of bearing witness.

Unless we name it, no one will know. Unless we speak it, no one will see.

A Culture That Keeps Us Quiet

We teach physicians to be resilient. To keep going. To compartmentalize. To endure.

After all, when a code blue does happen, we can't grieve or process. We go on to the next.

We rarely teach them how to speak up. Or slow down. Or ask for help. And so we build a culture of competent silence. Where suffering is managed with productivity. Where pain is buried beneath professionalism. Where a colleague can work next to you for years, while falling apart inside.

The Lesson He Left

He taught me that kindness can be a mask. That the most dependable people may be the most exhausted. That no one — no one — is immune from breaking.

I don't know what it would have taken to save him.

But I do know this:

We have to start making space for truth.

We have to normalize asking, "Are you really okay?"

We have to believe someone when they say, "I'm not."

We have to stop rewarding silence with praise.

And we have to remind each other that being human is not a liability — it is the beginning of healing.

Closing Thought

Behind every calm face may live a storm.

Behind every chart note may live a cry.

Behind every "fine" may live a fracture.

Let's not wait for the obituary to wonder what could have been done.

Let's notice each other — really notice.

Let's lead with presence, not assumptions.

Let's speak out before the next quiet collapse.

Because if medicine is truly about healing, **we must start with our own.**

CHAPTER 8

The One Who Heard It

Lesson: Nurses are closest to patients at their most vulnerable
— and when we listen to them, we save lives.

HE WAS 51 YEARS OLD. Admitted for confusion, fatigue, and vague abdominal discomfort. His vitals were stable. The labs were inconclusive. The imaging was unrevealing. I reviewed his chart three times, trying to find the missing piece.

He didn't make sense. Not yet.

He answered questions, but his affect was flat. His electrolytes were borderline but not critical. His liver enzymes mildly elevated. His CT scan showed nonspecific fullness of the abdomen. We ruled out infection, mass, bleeding. His mental status was "intact but slowed," according to the note I wrote. We ordered more tests. We waited. We watched.

But something didn't feel right.

And then the nurse came to find me.

The Most Important Detail

"I was in the room when his wife called," she said. "I had him on speakerphone because he was struggling to hold the phone. She mentioned something about a memory problem a few months ago ... and that he got really confused after eating shellfish. Has anyone looked into that?"

I paused.

Shellfish?

I hadn't asked about food allergies. It wasn't in the chart. No documentation. No classic anaphylaxis. But something in what she said stuck.

I went back and talked to the wife. She confirmed it. "Yeah, a couple of times he got really out of it after seafood. Not hives or anything. Just ... off."

The nurse had caught it — not just the words, but the meaning.

I re-reviewed the labs. Subtle eosinophilia. Abdominal pain. Cognitive changes. Something clicked.

I called for further allergy and immunology input. They suggested a rare condition — eosinophilic gastroenteritis, potentially food-triggered. Biopsy later confirmed it.

Treatment started. He improved.

Nurses Know the Story

That detail wasn't in the chart. It wasn't in my questions. It didn't come from a textbook. It came from a nurse listening — not just to the patient, but to their world. Their environment. Their story.

She wasn't trying to solve the case. She was just present. She caught what I missed.

This has happened more times than I can count.

And it's why I listen — always — to nurses.

Because nurses are there.

They are there when patients cry, when they whisper confessions, when they remember the one detail that changes the trajectory. They are there at night, at shift change, at the bedside for hours — not minutes. They see the progression. They feel the subtle shifts. They witness the unraveling long before we do.

They know when the pattern is off — even if they can't name the reason.

I Learned This Early

During residency, I would often stay on the wards long after my shift ended — not to chase procedures or impress anyone, but to listen. I'd sit at the nurse's station, quietly absorbing what they said and how they said it. I learned about patients in ways no note could capture. I learned to ask better questions. I learned to observe.

And the truth is: a nurse saved me.

A nurse saved me in medical school when I was drowning in self-doubt and didn't yet know how to lead.

A nurse saved me in residency when a patient's rapid change in status wasn't caught by vitals but by her intuition.

A nurse saved me as a new attending when I was about to make the wrong call and she gently redirected me.

And they save me still — every day.

The insight they have. The compassion they hold. The presence they embody. It is awe-inspiring.

Be humble to the nurses. Be curious to learn from them.

The healthcare team is everyone. Listen to your team — everyone. Be it a nurse, a new doctor, environmental services, social work, respiratory, physical therapy — anyone. You never know who will give you the one piece of information that changes everything for the person you are trying to save.

I Am Not Strong Enough to Be a Nurse

There is a strength in nursing I have always admired, but never claimed.

The strength to be present through bodily fluids, spiritual distress, and emotional unraveling — without flinching.

The strength to keep showing up during double shifts and short staffing.

The strength to comfort a patient who just got bad news, even when no one else knows yet.

The strength to know when to call for help — not out of fear, but from intuition.

I've learned more about patient care from nurses than I have from most medical textbooks.

Because I listened when I was documenting.

Because I stayed quiet when they shared a gut feeling.

Because I paid attention when they paused at the door, hesitant to leave.

Their wisdom is quiet. Humble. Often unrecognized.

But I can say with complete honesty: I have saved lives because I listened to nurses.

Reflection

Medical illness is often a detective story. The clues are rarely obvious. The labs may be normal. The images may be clean. But the truth hides in the most mundane detail — a word, a moment, a story told by a spouse, overheard in the early morning hours.

And nurses are the ones who catch it. Not always. Not every time. But more than we know. They will not always tell you what to do. But if you are humble enough to listen, they will give you what you need to see the bigger picture.

To Nurses, I Thank You

For the courage to speak up when it's easier to stay silent.

For the presence you bring when the rest of us are moving too fast.

For being the eyes, ears, and heart of the hospital.

For teaching me — quietly, patiently, and without needing recognition.

This chapter is for you.

This life saved is because of you.

And every day, I am a better doctor — because I listened.

CHAPTER 9

At the Table or on the Menu

Lesson: Leadership is presence. It is not about control,
but about clarity — especially when facing loss. We must
remain engaged in our own care and decisions.

HE WAS ALREADY SEATED WHEN I WALKED IN — upright in his power wheelchair, thin but sharp-eyed, with a quiet presence that filled the room before he spoke a word. He was 72, a retired physician and serial entrepreneur.

Though ALS had taken much of his strength, his presence was still commanding. I introduced myself, but I knew he already knew who I was. He had reviewed the staff list, read my bio, and made sure I was the attending scheduled to follow him.

He was a man who led from the front — even in illness.

He had been diagnosed with pancreatic cancer at age 64. A death sentence for many. But not for him. He underwent a Whipple procedure, followed by months of chemotherapy. He lost weight, lost muscle, lost time — but he never lost focus. He survived it. And when he emerged from that illness, he didn't slow down. He doubled down on life.

He returned to the businesses he had built, stayed active in his medical community, and more than anything, dedicated himself to caring for his wife, who had become gravely ill in his absence.

She had heart failure, end-stage renal disease, and required dialysis multiple times per week. He bathed her. Advocated for her. Coordinated her medications. He remained present as her partner and caregiver, even as he began to notice something unsettling in himself: muscle twitches, subtle weakness, then eventually slurred speech.

At age 69, he was diagnosed with ALS.

He didn't panic. He planned.

As the disease progressed — slowly at first — he adapted. He learned to use assistive technology. Modified his home. Dictated emails and policies through eye-tracking software. Even as he lost the ability to walk, then move his arms, then eat, he remained at the center of every conversation. He did not allow his disease to remove him from the table.

When his wife could no longer tolerate dialysis, he supported her decision to transition to hospice. He held her hand as she died. And I watched him — unable to speak without a voice amplifier, unable to move unaided — still command respect, still lead his care team, still teach.

When he told me he wanted to pursue Medical Assistance in Dying (MAID), he did not ask permission.

He told me plainly, through the speech device mounted to his wheelchair, "This is not about giving up. It's about choosing how I continue to lead my life — including how I leave it."

There was controversy, of course. Family members struggled with the idea. Friends resisted. Some staff had unspoken discomfort. But he invited everyone to the table. Not just to inform them, but to help them understand. He shared his reasons, his fears, and his faith in the decision.

One day during rounds, he told me something that would stay with me far beyond that unit, beyond that season of life:

"If you're not at the table, you're on the menu."

He said it with a wry smile, but he meant it. In healthcare. In business. In family. In life. Stay engaged, or someone else will make your decisions for you. His message wasn't just about medical autonomy. It was about *ownership*. About staying awake in your life, no matter what you've lost.

Reflection: What He Taught Me

I've met many leaders, but few like him. He showed me that leadership is not about power — it's about presence. It's about continuing to *be at the table*, even when everything in your body tells you to retreat. His clarity, even in the face of physical decline, taught me more about integrity than any lecture or leadership seminar ever could.

His choice to pursue MAID changed me.

Before meeting him, I had mixed feelings. I saw it as ethically complex, emotionally loaded, legally difficult. But he helped me see something different: that bravery doesn't always look like a fight. Sometimes, it looks like a deliberate step forward into the unknown — with your eyes open, your heart steady, and your values intact.

He wasn't choosing death. He was choosing *dignity*. He was choosing to remain the author of his life until the very last sentence.

And he gave that same clarity to those around him — his children, his caregivers, his colleagues, and me.

Closing Thought

He showed me that leadership isn't about what you command; it's about how you choose, how you stay present, and how you face even the hardest truths with clarity.

His life — and his death — reminded me that the most powerful form of leadership begins with owning your place at the table.

And his words guide me still:

If you're not at the table, you're on the menu.

Part III

Continuing *to* Care

∞

**Where clarity deepens, meaning returns,
and the work becomes a calling.**

CHAPTER 10

What Comes Next?

Lesson: Death is full of mystery, but in the final moments of life, patterns emerge that point to something greater. Patients often speak of seeing loved ones who've passed. These moments — regardless of belief — offer a kind of hope. Perhaps we are not alone at the end. Perhaps, even in death, we are accompanied.

HE WAS 91 YEARS OLD. A Korean War veteran. A man who had outlived his wife, all of his friends, and just recently, his dog, Skip.

He lived alone on his ranch, far enough outside of town that grocery trips were intentional. He was self-sufficient, proud, and until just a few months before I met him, still went on walks every morning.

He wasn't a gourmet cook, but he loved making simple meals. He said he cooked for Skip more than himself. Skip didn't mind. Skip loved people, loved other animals, and most of all, he loved his owner.

But over the last year, everything in the man's world had started to shrink —his appetite, his routines, his energy.

It started after his last close friend passed away. Without someone to talk to, he stopped making small trips into town. He no longer lingered at the diner. He stopped talking as much. The walks became shorter until they stopped altogether. The TV stayed on more — Matlock, The A-Team, the Giants no matter how badly they played — but it stopped being something he watched and became something that simply filled the space.

Skip passed away not long before his last admission to the hospital.

The human body is miraculous in its design — but it is also subject to the quiet laws of aging. As he ate less, his stomach adjusted. His muscles began to atrophy. As he stopped moving, his strength vanished more quickly. And when he did eat, the food no longer tasted the same. Too salty. Not salty enough. Too sweet. No sweetness at all.

Eventually, his swallow reflex weakened. He started to aspirate.

His first admission was for pneumonia. Then another. And another. Each time, he recovered just enough to go back home. But each time, he left a little less whole than before.

The last time he came in, I could see it in his eyes. His dog was gone. His friends were gone. The reason to keep going had dimmed.

And then came the Super Bowl.

His Giants were playing — a rare victory in itself. Normally, he would've been glued to the screen, yelling at the refs and mumbling about "the good old days." But that night, he just lay there, half-watching.

I pulled up a chair and sat with him. We watched in silence. Not because there was nothing to say, but because the ritual of sitting beside someone, watching something they love, was the only medicine I could offer.

The next morning, I stopped by his room.

He looked sharper. His eyes were clearer. There was a flicker of something I hadn't seen in days.

I sat down in the same chair I had used the night before.

"No!" he suddenly said, voice stronger than I expected. "Don't sit there!"

I froze, startled.

"Skip's mad at you."

He was serious. Not agitated. Not confused. Just... certain.

I paused. Then nodded.

"I'm sorry, Skip," I said. "Didn't mean to take your spot."

He relaxed again.

That afternoon, he died. Peacefully. Quietly. Alone — but not really.

What I've Seen Too Often to Ignore

That wasn't the first time I've seen something like that. And it wouldn't be the last.

Over the years, I've watched many people in their final days. I've witnessed a pattern I can't fully explain. People of every age, background, and belief system often speak to loved ones who've passed. They see them. Hear them. Feel their presence.

Sometimes it's a spouse. Sometimes a parent. Sometimes a child.

Or, in this case, a dog.

They talk to them like they're in the room. They reach toward them. They smile at them.

Science might call these hallucinations. And maybe, technically, they are. But when I see the peace that comes over someone who sees a familiar face near the end — whether it's real, imagined, or something else — I no longer try to label it.

Because what I do see is this: The fear fades. The tension leaves their face. They feel… accompanied.

And maybe that's what matters most.

Reflection: What Comes Next?

I've watched hundreds of people take their final breaths.

Some go suddenly. Some drift over days.

But in those last moments, when the monitors are silent, when the room is still, when there are no more questions to answer, there's often something else that arrives.

Not fear. Not confusion.

Something else. Something I can't measure or diagnose.

Something that looks a lot like love.

I don't know what happens when we die.

But if what I've seen is any indication, I have hope that we are not alone.

That we are met by the ones we loved, and perhaps even by the ones who loved us most.

Closing Thought

We spend so much of our time in medicine trying to fight death, delay it, redefine it. But what if part of our work is simply to witness it? To hold space for it — not with answers, but with presence?

In the end, we may not know what happens after this life. But I've come to believe that the final moments people experience are not random. They are patterned, familiar, sometimes astonishing.

And maybe that's the lesson: that death, like life, is not something we must walk through alone.

If we pay attention — not just to the labs, the vitals, or the protocols — but to the stories, the silences, and the soft goodbyes, we may find that dying is not the end of connection. It's another doorway into something we don't yet understand — but may not need to fear.

And in that space, there is room for hope.

CHAPTER 11

The Two-Hour Window

*Lesson: Even meaningful work can steal our time for health,
connection, and reflection. Our mind, body, and spirit
need daily attention — or we drift into imbalance.*

SHE CAME TO SEE ME FOR HELP WITH WEIGHT LOSS.

She was 38, an attorney with a high-powered job, a sharp intellect, and a voice that carried both precision and fatigue. Her schedule was packed. Her life, on paper, looked like a success story. But she didn't feel well. She told me, bluntly, "I'm just tired of feeling this way."

As we spoke, I learned that her story didn't begin in a courtroom.

It began on the field.

From Athlete to Advocate

In high school, she had been a three-season athlete. Cross country in the fall. Basketball in the winter. Tennis in the spring. She was also a straight-A student, in student government, and a Peer Leader. She had plans to go to medical school. Her life was organized around excellence — academic, athletic, and interpersonal.

Then came the injuries.

At 13, she tore her ACL playing tennis. Surgery and rehab followed. She returned to sport.

At 15, it happened again. Basketball.

At 19 — again. Tennis.

At 22 — again. Golf.

Each tear was more than a physical setback. It became a personal reckoning. Her body kept failing her, and slowly, her confidence followed. By the time she was 21, she was close to failing out of college. She had gained weight. She stopped moving. She became disconnected — from sport, from study, from herself.

46

At 13, she had weighed 85 pounds. By the time she graduated, she was 280.

She still graduated pre-med, but her GPA couldn't get her into medical school. She drifted — uncertain, disheartened. She took a job at a friend's law firm.

And then, a moment.

One day, after helping with a complicated case, the lawyer she worked for looked at her and said, "You would make an excellent attorney."

That was enough.

She applied. She got in. And she found her path.

Success, With a Cost

She became a successful lawyer. Smart, thorough, respected. But the habits that had once grounded her — movement, nutrition, rest — were long gone.

She had no major vices. She didn't smoke, didn't drink excessively. But she ate quickly, slept poorly, and rarely moved. Her weight peaked at 310 pounds. She had tried every diet, every program. She could lose 40–50 pounds. But it always came back.

That's when we met.

She didn't need another crash diet. She needed a new rhythm.

The Set Point Trap

The body remembers its heaviest weight.

Once your physiology sets a new "normal," it fights to maintain it. The brain regulates appetite, metabolism, and cravings to defend this set point. That's why restrictive diets often fail long-term.

She had lived through that cycle for years.

What she needed was integration — not punishment.

We worked on sleep first. Then food. Then movement.

Not all at once, but in manageable layers.

The science was clear: To maintain lost weight and avoid regain, a person needs 45–60 minutes of daily exercise, every single day.

But she worked 12 hours. Her commute was 2. She needed 8 hours of sleep.

That left her two hours to do everything else in life: eat, move, connect, breathe.

How could she possibly make room?

The Answer Was: She Did

Slowly, she found her rhythm.

She made meals simpler and more deliberate. Ate slower. Ate less. Chose foods that nourished her. She got a standing desk. Started walking calls. Began stretching before bed. Prioritized movement — not all at once, but as a thread woven into her day.

She didn't chase perfection. She practiced presence.

The weight came down — from 310 to 125.

And this time, it stayed off.

Reflection: What She Taught Me

This patient taught me that we professionals often sacrifice our health in the name of purpose. We love what we do. We believe it matters. But without care, that same purpose can consume the time and energy we owe to our own lives.

We must give the mind space to learn — but also to cool down.

We must move our bodies — not just for weight, but for vitality.

We must feed our spirits — with laughter, connection, stillness, and love.

If we don't, our lives become one-dimensional — successful, perhaps, but incomplete.

She reminded me that a full life isn't built in grand gestures. It's built in the two-hour window we fight to protect. The one that matters more than the meeting, the inbox, or the metrics.

We have to live lives we'd be proud to return to — not just careers we're proud to climb.

Closing Thought

We are not machines. We are human.

And even when our work is meaningful, we still need movement. We need quiet. We need joy.

If we don't build habits to protect those needs, the work will take every bit of space we give it.

This patient taught me that the difference between surviving and flourishing is often found not in the hours we work — but in the hours we keep for ourselves.

CHAPTER 12

Keep Moving Forward

Lesson: Life will get hijacked. But we still have a choice:
to move forward. One step, one breath, one act of courage at a time.

She told me once, calmly and without complaint:

"Even if my life gets hijacked, I'm going to keep moving forward. For my kids. For my patients. For myself."

She wasn't trying to inspire me when she said it. It was simply her truth.

She was 58. A physician. A mother of two. A woman who had endured more than most people will ever face — and yet every time I saw her, she met me with clarity, resilience, and a quiet steadiness that never wavered.

The Weight She Carried

She was first diagnosed with cervical cancer when she was 38. It was a life-altering moment, but she got through it — surgery, treatment, recovery. She returned to work, returned to her life, kept going.

Not long after came another blow: breast cancer.

This time it was tougher — chemotherapy, radiation, and surgery. Her hair fell out. Her strength declined. But she endured it all with the same steady focus.

She went into remission. Again, she got back to life. Again, she moved forward.

By the time I began caring for her, she was experiencing symptoms of heart failure. We eventually diagnosed restrictive cardiomyopathy, a consequence of Alpha-1 antitrypsin deficiency, compounded by the long-term effects of her cancer treatments. Her breathing was becoming more difficult. Her body was tired.

But her spirit remained undiminished.

A Mother, a Doctor, a Survivor

She had two children.

Her first pregnancy ended in an emergency C-section after she developed severe preeclampsia. It was traumatic — physically and emotionally — but she never saw herself as fragile. She saw herself as fortunate. Her baby lived.

Her second child was born via scheduled C-section. This child would later be diagnosed with developmental delays. She met that challenge with the same grit she had met all the others.

She balanced parenting, caregiving, and her medical career — always with humility, never with complaint.

And then came the greatest loss of all: her husband.

He was diagnosed with pancreatic cancer at just 44. He died at 46.

She was a widow at 48. A single mother. A physician still practicing. And now, once again, a patient.

Showing Up Anyway

Despite it all, she kept working.

She kept mothering.

She kept mentoring.

There were days when her legs swelled, her breathing grew shallow, her fatigue crept in like a fog. But she showed up — for her patients, for her kids, for herself.

She had no illusions. She knew the limits of her body. But she refused to surrender her life to them.

She told me once, "I know how fragile it all is. But as long as I can still give something, I'm going to keep giving."

The Lesson She Taught Me

Strength is often quiet.

It's not in the speeches or the stories we post online — it's in the people who keep going when no one's watching. Who wake up, dress, and care when they themselves are barely held together.

She showed me that grit isn't a personality trait. It's a choice.

And perseverance isn't about pretending things are okay. It's about choosing to keep moving anyway.

Reflection

She taught me that medicine is not only about curing — it's about walking beside.

I didn't fix her. I couldn't. But I witnessed her. I supported her. I reminded her that she didn't have to carry it alone.

And in doing so, I learned how to carry my own burdens with more grace.

Her life was not easy. Her path was not fair. But she never let adversity define her.

She chose to live with purpose, even as the world kept trying to take that choice away.

Closing Thought

We all get hijacked.

By diagnoses. By grief. By loss. By uncertainty.

But we don't have to stop.

We can move forward. Not because it's easy. Not because it's fair. But because we are still here.

And sometimes, that's reason enough.

Part IV

Algorithms *of* Care

∞

**Where technology meets presence — and
the future of medicine is at stake.**

CHAPTER 13

When the Algorithm
Got It Wrong

Lesson: Algorithms can enhance care, but overreliance on them without clinical judgment can lead to harm. The erosion of history-taking and physical exam as core tools is a quiet crisis. Premature diagnostic closure is dangerous in human practice — and catastrophic when coded into machines without an understanding of clinical nuance.

The alert came before the patient.

"Sepsis suspected. CODE Sepsis paged overhead. Protocol initiated. Broad-spectrum antibiotics. Three-liter bolus. Stat labs drawn. CXR flagged with possible right lower lobe consolidation. Vital signs outside parameters."

It was all there, presented in a clean, linear digital narrative: everything the algorithm needed to determine urgency, risk, and the next steps. I had not yet spoken to the patient or family. I hadn't even heard the sound of his breathing. But the chart was already a story, and the story was sepsis.

He was 82. Brought in by his daughter who had noticed he was more tired, more breathless, and acting "a little off." EMS had started oxygen. His lactate was mildly elevated. His heart rate crept into the triple digits. The chest X-ray, flagged by our AI-assisted imaging system, suggested pneumonia. The orders populated automatically, built off what we now call "decision support." In truth, they were decisions already made.

By the time I reached him, a nurse was finishing the third liter of IV fluids.

He looked pale, but not flushed. His breathing was labored, but not rapid. He spoke in short phrases, and I caught the distinct cadence of someone struggling not because of infection, but because of fluid.

His extremities were cool. His neck veins, barely visible with him reclined, became distended when I raised the head of the bed. He had bilateral crackles — not focal, not patchy — and a third heart sound I almost missed beneath the hiss of nasal cannula flow. There was no fever. No rigors.

No cough. His white count was normal. The infiltrate? Likely vascular congestion.

And the antibiotics? The fluids? They were wrong.

He didn't need more volume. He needed less. What he was drowning in was not infection — but us.

I ordered furosemide and discontinued the fluids. Hours later, his breathing eased. By morning, he looked like a different person.

But I didn't feel victorious. I felt shaken.

I had almost missed it.

Not because I didn't know what CHF looked like — but because I had almost trusted the system more than I trusted myself.

This is Not a Story of Blame

It's a story of drift.

We are drifting away from the bedside. Away from the patient's story, and toward the screen. Protocols replace presence. AI replaces inquiry. What once started as a tool has quietly become a crutch.

The initial misdiagnosis was not malicious. It was systemic. It was a result of a workflow that prioritizes rapid triage and checkbox medicine. And it made sense — on paper. Elevated heart rate? Low oxygen? Infiltrate on chest X-ray? The algorithm is trained to act. But the context was wrong.

We as physicians were trained differently once. History and physical exam were not just formality — they were the essence of diagnosis. But today, how often is a full exam deferred? How often is the history outsourced to a nurse's triage note or a family member's voicemail? It is faster to click. It is more efficient to accept the alert.

But faster is not wiser.

The Greater Risk

If these algorithmic shortcuts are used to build the next generation of artificial intelligence, then the AI will not just inherit our errors — it will amplify them. Flawed clinical pathways will become hardcoded logic.

Heuristics will become gospel. And the art of medicine will be buried beneath the confidence of the machine.

Premature closure — a well-known cognitive error in clinical reasoning — occurs when we settle on a diagnosis too soon, ignoring or misinterpreting data that doesn't fit. When this kind of error becomes embedded in the training of an AI system, it becomes something far more insidious: systematic, scalable misdiagnosis. The AI doesn't second-guess. It doesn't hesitate. It acts with the certainty of code — and without the humility of doubt.

It doesn't learn empathy. It doesn't ask follow-up questions. It doesn't notice the subtle hesitation in a family member's voice. It doesn't place a hand on a swollen leg or listen for the cadence of rales across a chest. It learns from data — and if the data rewards speed over nuance, code over compassion, it will carry those values forward.

But Medicine Is Not Binary

It is breath, and texture, and silence. It is shaped not only by what is said, but by how it is said. And these truths are not in the algorithm. They are at the bedside.

That patient did well. We stopped the fluids. Started diuretics. Within 24 hours, his breathing eased and the fog lifted from his mind. But I was haunted by how close we came to harming him. Not from neglect — but from trust. Trust in a system designed for speed, not understanding.

Reflection

As physicians, we must reclaim the centrality of our role — not just as interpreters of data, but as stewards of human stories. The history and physical exam remain the most powerful tools we have. They cost nothing. They reveal everything.

We must also recognize our own cognitive vulnerabilities — and be vigilant not to hardwire them into the systems we build. Because what we teach AI is not just medicine — it is our mindset.

Let us not forget how to listen. Let us not forget how to see.

Let us not forget how to be — present, human, fallible, and awake — in the sacred space between heartbeats.

Closing Thought

If we allow algorithms to replace inquiry, and protocols to replace presence, we risk becoming observers of a system rather than participants in a healing relationship.

AI can be a tool. But it must never become the storyteller. That role belongs to the patient — and it is our responsibility to listen.

Because what saves lives is not just the data we collect, but the meaning we make from it.

And the meaning still lives — between heartbeats.

CHAPTER 14

One Algorithm Said No, Another Said Yes

Lesson: AI-driven decisions about inpatient status and reimbursement risk distorting care, minimizing physician judgment, and making patients invisible to the system.

SHE WAS 79. FRAIL BUT FIERCELY INDEPENDENT. Her daughter wheeled her into the emergency room, worried about increasing weakness and shortness of breath.

"She's not herself," the daughter said. "She's barely eating, can't stand up, and seems confused."

From the doorway, the patient looked stable — quiet, upright in the chair, breathing with some effort but not gasping. But when I stepped closer, I saw the signs: dry mucous membranes, postural hypotension, bibasilar crackles, shallow respirations, and an undercurrent of fatigue that suggested far more than "just deconditioning."

We ran the labs. Her creatinine was elevated. Chest imaging was equivocal. She had borderline vitals but no overt source of infection. In the real world, this was a patient we admit — monitor closely, correct her fluid status, prevent complications, and get her strength back under supervision.

But a call from the insurance company said she did not qualify for an inpatient stay. Their AI algorithm had reviewed her chart and concluded she could be managed as an outpatient. She was sick enough to be hospitalized, and we were treating her — but to the algorithm, the documentation did not justify the expense.

And that's what it comes down to: expense, not care.

The Algorithms Said No

The algorithms used to determine whether the patient should be classified as inpatient or outpatient said no.

According to their automated logic, she didn't meet inpatient criteria. But that determination didn't just influence where she was labeled in the EMR — it influenced what she would owe. If she were categorized as outpatient observation, her coverage would shift. She would be responsible for a significantly higher out-of-pocket cost — for medically necessary care.

This is the part of modern medicine that few patients ever see. An invisible hand deciding what is reimbursed — and therefore, what is possible.

The Peer-to-Peer

On the other end was a medical director from the insurance company. Pleasant. Detached. Reading from a script.

But this wasn't just a conversation. This was a ritual of resistance. The gatekeeping protocol of a system that no longer trusts the judgment of the provider at the bedside.

The insurance company had developed its own AI, trained on years of claims data, rejections, and documentation triggers. It wasn't built to understand care. It was built to find reasons to deny it.

So I fought back — with the same tools.

Using our HIPAA-compliant AI assistant, I mined the EMR for what mattered: vital signs, documented decline, home support gaps, comorbidities, fall risk. I synthesized the evidence into a coherent story — one that could stand up to algorithmic scrutiny.

Because today, documentation isn't just for continuity. It's for defense.

The AI helped me make the case. I argued not just from clinical sense but from system-savvy language. The peer reviewer agreed. Her inpatient status was approved. Her care would be covered. Her outcome, protected.

When Documentation Becomes Defense

That night, I realized something unsettling.

We are no longer documenting to tell the truth. We are documenting to match a formula.

The physician's note is now parsed by machines trained to look for billable terms. Not insights. Not context. Not judgment. If you don't say "acute hypoxic respiratory failure," if you forget to mention "frailty index," if you miss the phrase "risk of rapid deterioration" — then the care doesn't count.

The risk is not just denial. It is distortion.

Real medicine is being rewritten by the logic of billing algorithms. And slowly, clinicians are being trained — without realizing it — to write for compliance instead of clarity. To code, not to communicate.

As intermediaries multiply in healthcare — coders, payers, auditors, insurance, PBMs, and now algorithms — the distance between patient and provider grows. Each added layer introduces complexity that must be paid for. And what pays for it? A single interaction: between a patient and the provider trying to help them. That moment is now parsed, scored, and reimbursed by logic written for systems, not stories.

A Battle of Bots

Maybe someday we'll see AI systems trained to defend care as precisely as others are built to deny it.

A physician's AI that understands nuance. That integrates social factors. That flags unspoken risks. That advocates the way we once did — with language, presence, and clinical intuition.

But then we'll have bot versus bot. An automated audit against an automated appeal. A war of scripts while the patient lies quietly in bed, waiting for one side to win.

And we'll call this progress.

But I don't want to win the documentation war. I want to win the patient back to health.

The Broader Hijack

This story is not just about algorithms. It's about a system hijacked.

As more intermediaries entered healthcare — administrators, payers, IT vendors, coders, consultants — the complexity ballooned. Every layer demanded justification. Every justification required documentation. Every documentation created jobs. Every job required funding. And the source of that funding? The original act of care between one patient and one provider.

So we built protocols to distill it. Then came AI to interpret it. And now we have software that decides, often without understanding, whether care is "valid."

Physicians, in ceding the knowledge of how care is delivered and paid for, allowed this to happen. By stepping back from system design, from process improvement, from management, we surrendered our seat at the table.

Now, more than ever, we must reclaim it.

We must understand not only the science of healing, but the machinery of healthcare. We must become leaders — not just in treatment, but in advocacy.

Because if we don't understand the system, we cannot fix it. And if we cannot fix it, our patients will pay for that ignorance with their health — and their savings.

Closing Thought

The woman I fought for recovered. She left the hospital five days later, steadier, stronger, and smiling. Her daughter hugged me and said, "Thank you for taking her seriously."

But I couldn't shake the question: **What if I hadn't fought? What if the computer's "no" had been final?**

There is a quiet erosion happening in healthcare. It doesn't crash. It doesn't scream. It hums in the background — rewriting care in the language of codes and costs.

If we want AI to support us, it must be built to amplify care, not obscure it. Because when the algorithm says no, it still must be the physician who says yes — when it matters most.

And it does matter.

Healthcare providers will need to learn methods to process information and narrate a story that advocates for the person they are trying to heal.

When physicians took a back seat in the management of healthcare, we allowed this to happen. Now more than ever, we need to learn about how healthcare is delivered, how it is paid for, how to process-improve, and how to manage.

We must earn our seat at the table and advocate for the people we care for. Because at the heart of every system, buried beneath the workflows and workflows-about-workflows, is a single, sacred moment: **One patient. One provider. One chance to heal.**

CHAPTER 15

Finding Her Story Again

*Lesson: When used with intention, AI can
help us connect a fragmented system.*

SHE WAS 82, WHEELED INTO OUR NURSING home late on a rainy Thursday afternoon. The transfer summary was sparse — two typed paragraphs and a med list. The admitting note from the sending facility was generic. No clear goals of care. No history of what led her here. Just another transition in a long, fragmented journey.

Her name was Mrs. M. And at first glance, she looked tired. Thin. Her hands were tremulous. She wore a faint look of resignation — the kind of expression patients carry after being passed between hospitals, rehabs, and nursing homes for too long.

There was a moment — one that's become all too familiar — where I felt a familiar frustration rise: *How am I supposed to make good decisions for her if I can't even find her story?*

In the past, I would've spent the next hour clicking through disconnected notes, scouring hospital portals, calling outside facilities, waiting on faxed records, and trying to reverse-engineer her past through guesswork.

But this time was different.

This time, I had help.

The Tools That Listened

I activated the ambient AI tool as I sat down with Mrs. M. It recorded our conversation, identifying my questions, her responses, the physical exam, the plan, and even the nuanced tone of our interaction. While I spoke with her — fully, attentively — it quietly documented in the background. Not word-for-word, but meaning-for-meaning.

Then I turned to the large language model integrated with our health information exchange. With a single request, it retrieved and summarized two years of care across four hospital admissions, three skilled nursing facility stays, and countless outpatient visits.

Instead of 30 PDFs and disconnected portal logins, I had a timeline. A story.

What I Learned

She had suffered a pelvic fracture two years prior after a fall on ice. She'd been hospitalized three times for infections — one of which resulted in sepsis and a prolonged ICU stay. She had completed rehab twice but regressed both times after being discharged too soon. She had been read-mitted for a TIA. Her dementia had worsened after each hospitalization. She had undergone two rounds of chemotherapy for lymphoma but had missed follow-up due to transportation barriers.

None of this was in the transfer note.

But it was all there — buried in scanned progress notes, discharge summaries, and prior H&Ps across the region.

The AI summarized it in three paragraphs, followed by links to every source.

The Encounter That Mattered

Because I had the context, I didn't need to spend our encounter checking boxes. I spent it talking with her.

I asked her what she remembered about her illness. She told me about the fall that started it all. How she had once been active, independent, cooking every night, and walking to church. How she started to lose pieces of herself after each hospital stay. How she missed her garden.

She didn't remember every diagnosis. But she remembered the grief of losing her old life.

Because I knew her story, I didn't ask irrelevant questions. I didn't repeat labs. I didn't put her through another CT scan "just to be sure." I talked to her about what she wanted next. What quality of life looked like now. Whether she felt safe. And what she feared most.

And I had time to do it.

Because I wasn't buried in the chart.

I wasn't scrolling through PDFs.

I wasn't recreating work that had already been done.

I was present.

What It Gave Back

Documentation fatigue is real. It creeps in not only as exhaustion, but as disconnection. We start to document to satisfy billing, not to understand. To survive, not to remember.

But this encounter reminded me that when used intentionally, AI can give us something back: time.

Time to be a doctor again. Time to listen. Time to think.

Ambient AI wrote the bulk of my note. The LLM pulled the records and organized them. All I did was review, refine, and re-engage.

The patient may not have realized that technology was working in the background. But she knew that I was fully there — with her. And that made all the difference.

Reflection

We often speak of AI as a threat to the human elements of care. And in some cases, it can be. But if we design it right — if we guide its use — AI can be a bridge back to presence.

It can free us from the tyranny of the inbox. From the endless clicking. From the documentation treadmill that steals our evenings and shortens our patience.

It can help us reclaim what we never should have lost: time with our patients. Context for our decisions. And the quiet satisfaction of *knowing someone's story before we try to change it.*

Closing Thought

Mrs. M reminded me that people don't arrive as "new patients." They arrive carrying history — some of it spoken, much of it buried in systems not designed to be read by humans.

When the record is scattered, we lose the thread. But when AI helps us find it again, we rediscover not only the patient — but ourselves.

Because when you see the story, you see the person.

And when you see the person, you know what to do.

And that — always — lives between heartbeats.

CHAPTER 16

The Journey Continues

Lesson: In an age where algorithms and systems threaten to standardize care, our greatest responsibility is to preserve the human heart of medicine — by showing up, staying present, and continuing to light the way for others.

WHEN I STARTED MEDICAL SCHOOL IN 2009, I didn't have a clear reason for becoming a physician. I didn't have a "why." I just had a sense that medicine was important — that it would matter.

Over time, that instinct matured. My "why" evolved into a desire to help people. Then it transformed again — into a deeper calling to learn people's stories, not just to understand them better, but to understand myself. I realized that by bearing witness to my patients' lives, their suffering, and their resilience, I could become a better physician — and a better human being.

Now, my purpose is to empower others through service and self-awareness.

To not only provide care, but to cultivate meaning.

That, for me, is the heart of medicine.

The Roles We Play

I feel incredibly lucky to be in a profession that allows me to be all of the following — sometimes in a single day:

- A detective, solving complex puzzles.
- A researcher, chasing truth.
- A lawyer, advocating fiercely.
- An entrepreneur, building new ways to serve.
- A technologist, embracing innovation.
- A student, always learning.
- A teacher, passing on what I've learned.
- A leader, making difficult decisions.
- A mediator, navigating human conflict.
- A mentor and coach, supporting the growth of others.

Few professions offer this kind of layered, evolving purpose.

Fewer still offer a front-row seat to the fullness of human life.

Medicine has given me that.

But we are at risk of losing this richness.

Preserving the Art

We are living through a time of tremendous change in healthcare. Data now drives decisions. Documentation guides reimbursement. AI systems are being trained to interpret, summarize, even respond.

Much of this is progress. But it comes with a cost.

The quiet parts of medicine — the parts where presence, intuition, and connection live — don't show up in billing codes. They're not tracked on dashboards. They're not considered "value-added." And yet, they are often the most valuable moments of all.

If we're not intentional, these moments will vanish. Replaced by standardized scripts. By decision trees. By prompts that say, "move on."

We can do better in healthcare.

An Evolving Why

There's a myth in medicine that you must start with a calling. But the truth is, your calling changes — just like you do.

Today, my "why" is this:

To learn through story, grow with purpose, and continually improve — so that I can empower others on their own journey of growth and meaning.

Restoring the Sacred Space

Where systems meet presence, and leadership becomes legacy.

In every clinical system, there are fractures — small and large — that separate the patient from the provider.

Paperwork replaces presence. Clicks replace conversation. Metrics measure everything — except what matters most.

The space between the clinician and the patient was once sacred. A place where trust was built, stories were shared, and healing began — not always with cures, but always with connection.

Today, that space is crowded.

EMRs fill the room. AI hovers overhead.

Payers, protocols, and policies layer into every encounter.

The provider types. The patient waits.

The moment slips away.

But the sacred space can be rebuilt.

Reclaiming Presence

Rebuilding that space does not mean rejecting technology.

It means anchoring it in human intention.

We don't need less efficiency — we need more humanity built into it.

- Ambient AI that listens while we do.
- EMR tools that capture meaning, not just codes.
- Shared documentation that reflects values, not just diagnoses.

At our hospital, we began integrating AI tools that work behind the scenes — drafting notes, pulling forward stories from the record, surfacing risks before they become problems.

But we also trained our clinicians to ask better questions.

To lead with, "What's most important to you today?"

To pause after a diagnosis and say, "Tell me what this means to you."

We paired innovation with intention.

Technology with presence.

And in doing so, we found a way to return to the work that matters most.

Healing the System from Within

Restoring the sacred space also means healing our culture.

That means rehumanizing leadership.

Creating spaces where nurses, aides, therapists, and physicians speak freely — and are heard.

It means investing in trauma-informed leadership, not just trauma-informed care.

Teaching humility, curiosity, and courage — not just clinical guidelines.

In my role, I've come to see systems not as cold mechanisms — but as ecosystems.

Places where values must be embedded in design.

Because our systems will only ever reflect the humanity we insist on.

A Legacy of Meaning

As physicians, we spend much of our lives reacting — to illness, to schedules, to change.

But part of leadership is choosing what to protect.

I want to protect the space between the question and the answer.

Between the note and the story.

Between the protocol and the person.

That is where healing lives.

That is where medicine still breathes.

That is the space worth restoring.

The Mirror and the Flame

Medicine is a mirror. It reflects who we are, and who we are becoming. But it also hands us a flame — a responsibility to carry our presence, compassion, and humanity into spaces that are often cold, clinical, and unforgiving.

If we are not careful, that flame will flicker and go out — under the weight of metrics, inboxes, and burnout.

But a candle only needs a spark, some wick, and oxygen to burn.

If we tend to our own flame — carefully, honestly, consistently — we can continue to light others.

Even now. Especially now.

Closing Thought

When I started this journey, I didn't know what kind of doctor I wanted to be.

Now I do.

I want to be the kind of doctor who remembers that a patient is a person.

Who values stories as much as studies.

Who sees presence not as optional, but as sacred.

In this age of the algorithm, preserving our humanity isn't nostalgic — it's necessary.

I am still walking. Still learning. Still lighting candles, wherever I can. And that, now more than ever, may be the most important work of all.

Because the sacred space doesn't disappear. It gets buried.

Under pressure. Under protocol. Under silence.

But it is still there — waiting.

To restore it is not just to fight for better care.

It is to reclaim the very reason we showed up in the first place.

And it is in that space — quiet, deliberate, human — **where the future of medicine will be written.**

Between heartbeats.

Epilogue

The Work That Remains

Medicine is changing.

It is faster. More efficient. More data-driven than ever before. Artificial intelligence is now reading charts, writing notes, assisting diagnoses, and measuring outcomes.

Healthcare has become more systematized, standardized, and algorithmically informed. And much of that has brought good.

But something sacred is being lost in the process. What's disappearing isn't science. It's soul. Not accuracy — but *intimacy*. Not outcomes — but *presence*.

As physicians, we are being asked to do more — with less.

To see faster, chart better, optimize throughput, and justify every action with a billing code. But the deepest truths I've learned in medicine didn't come from a dashboard or a data point. They came from sitting in silence with someone who was dying. From holding space for grief, confusion, and uncertainty — when there was nothing left to fix.

From moments no algorithm could predict, and no template could capture.

These are the parts of medicine that we cannot afford to lose.

We are told to focus on "value-added care."

But the most valuable care I've given has rarely been billable. It happened when I paused before a family meeting.

When I chose to listen longer than I had time for.

When I sat beside a patient and simply asked, *"What matters now?"* This book was born from those moments.

Moments when patients, often unknowingly, taught me how to stay human in a system that makes it easy to forget.

Moments that reminded me that even in the age of algorithms and metrics, there is still space for compassion, humility, and presence — if we choose to make room for it.

And so the work that remains is not just clinical. It is cultural. It is human.

We must protect the art of medicine.

We must teach presence as seriously as we teach pathophysiology. We must value listening — not just as a soft skill, but as a core act of healing. We must stay awake to what matters — especially now.

I am still walking this path.

Still asking the questions my patients asked me first.

Still learning how to be the kind of doctor — and person — I would want at my own bedside. I hope you are too.

Because in this age of the algorithm, preserving our humanity may be the most important work of all.

Prescriptions for Preserving Humanity in Healthcare

Practical reflections and strategies for those committed to healing, not just treating.

1. Protect the History and Physical Exam

The history and physical exam are not just tools for diagnosis — they are rituals of connection. At the bedside, trust is built through presence, not just results.

Action: Advocate for protected time during rounds and clinical encounters for hands-on examination and bedside teaching. Restore the physical exam as a therapeutic, humanizing act — not just a checkbox.

2. Reclaim the Patient Story

Documentation has become a battleground of metrics. But behind every checkbox is a life. The story is not noise — it is a signal.

Action: Teach narrative medicine. Encourage free-text summaries that honor the patient's voice. Build EMRs that capture context, not just codes. Actively listen to the patient, not to respond, but to just listen.

3. Train Human-Centered AI

AI must amplify judgment, not replace it. If we train algorithms only on what's billable or convenient, we risk hardcoding bias and losing the nuance that defines care.

Action: Involve frontline clinicians in the development, training, and oversight of healthcare AI. EMRs weren't designed with us in mind — let's not make that mistake again.

4. Acknowledge Collateral Damage

Every decision we make in healthcare — whether on the frontlines or behind the scenes — leaves a ripple. The burden of care can accumulate silently.

Action: Know your triggers. Learn your "tells." When disorganization creeps in or your energy wanes, take pause. Listen when a colleague asks, "Are you okay?" It may be the check-in that changes everything.

5. Redefine Value in Care

In LEAN methodology, value is defined by the customer. In medicine, that should be the patient — not the insurer, not the algorithm, not the litigation system.

Action: Advocate for payment models that reward time, complexity, continuity, and relationship-centered care. Reclaim value by remembering who we serve — and why.

6. Center Wellness as a Clinical Imperative

A burnt-out clinician cannot offer presence, creativity, or joy. Wellness is not a luxury — it is the foundation of sustainable, compassionate care.

Action: Institutionalize coaching, reflection, peer support, and recovery time as essential components of professional life — not optional add-ons.

7. Elevate the Voice of the Bedside

Too often, clinical decisions are made far from the patient. Policies are drafted without the stories that give them soul.

Action: Create formal structures for bedside clinicians, nurses, and families to inform quality initiatives and policy decisions. Be at the table. Advocate not just for outcomes — but for understanding.

8. Practice Trauma-Informed Care — Systemically

What we call "noncompliance" is often a story of protection. Trauma doesn't always announce itself — it hides in behavior we too easily judge.

Action: Train all staff in trauma-informed language, documentation, and care planning. Replace "noncompliant" with "barriers to adherence." Lead with curiosity, not control.

9. Lead with Humility. Stay with Grit.

Leadership is presence. It is listening, learning, and lifting others — especially when the room is hard, and the answers aren't clear.

Action: Schedule walkrounds not to inspect, but to connect. Ask, "What's one thing I can do to make your work easier?" Learn LEAN. Get leadership training from AAPL or SHM. Get a degree when it makes sense. But more importantly — be a follower before you lead.

10. Remember Why You Started

The system will challenge your purpose. Don't let it erase it.

Action: Create space to reflect. Weekly, monthly, daily — whatever it takes. Share stories. Reconnect with meaning. Keep the flame lit. Because at the heart of medicine, still and always, is one patient, one provider, one chance to heal.

A Letter to the Next Generation

To the medical students, residents, nurses, future clinicians, and all those walking toward a life of healing.

Dear Colleague,

You are entering medicine at a time of transformation.

The tools are smarter. The systems are faster. The algorithms are everywhere. The notes are templated. The decisions feel predetermined. It can be tempting to believe that your job is to comply, to click, to document, to follow the path someone else laid out for you.

But I need you to know something — something I didn't fully understand when I began this journey:

You are not a technician. You are not a cog in a billing machine. You are not defined by your efficiency.

You are a healer.

And healing happens in the space between protocols.

It lives in the moments that can't be measured — when you sit beside a patient in silence, when you ask a question no one else thought to ask, when you notice the tremble in a voice or the courage it takes to say, "I'm scared."

You will learn procedures. You will learn pharmacology, physiology, and pathology. You will learn how to admit, how to discharge, how to code, how to refer.

But never forget to learn how to see.

Because there will come a day when the labs don't explain the pain. When the chart is incomplete. When the algorithm says no, but your instincts say yes. In those moments, your presence will matter more than your precision.

And those are the moments that will stay with you.

This profession will stretch you.

It may exhaust you.

It may disappoint you.

But it will also give you access to the deepest parts of the human experience.

Grief. Hope. Birth. Death. Forgiveness. Resilience. Grace.

So here is my hope for you:

I hope you never lose your curiosity.

I hope you never chart so fast that you forget to ask, "What matters most to you right now?"

I hope you trust your judgment even when the system doesn't.

I hope you protect your own humanity — not just for yourself, but because your patients need it too.

And when the day comes — because it will — when you feel like stepping back, when you question whether you're making a difference, I hope you remember this:

You are enough.

Not because of what you do, but because of how you show up.

And showing up — fully, humbly, and with an open heart — is what will keep the flame alive.

We are counting on you — not just to carry medicine forward, but to carry it wisely.

With presence.

With integrity.

With love.

Between heartbeats,

— Devjit Roy

A Letter to My Wife and Children

There were days I came home with nothing left to give. Not because I didn't want to be with you, but because the work had taken everything from me. And I didn't always know how to say that. I wish I had.

There were weekends lost to call shifts, dinners interrupted by phone calls, decisions in leadership, and moments — precious ones — I'll never get back. You saw me look tired. Distant. Pulled into a world that felt invisible but urgent. And you never stopped loving me through it.

To my wife: I know this journey hasn't been easy. You've carried so much — more than I could ever measure — while I gave so much of myself to others. You held the family together in the quiet hours when I couldn't be there. You made room for my purpose, even when it meant sacrificing yours. And still, you smiled. Still, you stayed.

To my children: One day, you may wonder why I wasn't always present. I hope this book helps explain. The stories I write about here — the lives, the lessons, the heartbeats — taught me how to be a better doctor. But more importantly, they're teaching me how to be a better father. I am learning to be present, to listen, to slow down — because of you.

I wrote this book to preserve something sacred in medicine. But I also wrote it to honor you — my family. You are the reason I keep going. You are the reason I come back. And everything I am trying to protect out there — humanity, presence, purpose — I first learned with you.

I love you. I'm grateful for you. And I am sorry for the time you lost to the work I couldn't put down.

But I promise: I see it now. I see you.

And this book, in every word, is also a love letter home.

— DEV

www.ingramcontent.com/pod-product-compliance
Lightning Source LLC
Chambersburg PA
CBHW061837220326
41599CB00027B/5313